Royal Butterfly

Discover the Beauty Within

By

Debra L. O'Melia

ISBN: 1-4140-4239-6 (e-book)
ISBN: 1-4140-4240-X (Paperback)

This book is printed on acid free paper.

1stBooks - rev. 02/03/04

Dedication…..

To My Children Sean and Katelyn,

Who Have Given Me a Purpose and a Reason to Go On

Acknowledgments

With love and recognition to my son Sean for his talent, time and patience in helping me to prepare my manuscript for publication. To my friends and others that I hold dear, I thank you all so very much for always being there when I needed you, to share my laughter or endure my tears. To my "partners in fitness" who have been a source of encouragement, support and understanding, I send my appreciation and best wishes. To all the warm hearts that I have found on my way, I offer my gratitude for their care and fellowship. And most importantly, I give special affirmation to The One who watches over us all and who creates the beauty inside of everyone.

Table of Contents

Introduction

It is often said that a person has to walk the walk before they can talk the talk. Ten years ago the thought of writing a self-help book would have never entered my mind. Self-improvement was not on my list of priorities, even though I was in definite need of some positive changes in my life. What you'll read on these pages is my story about how I have dealt with some or the same problems that have plagued many overweight people. I'm not a doctor, celebrity or fitness wizard. I'm a woman who has spent a good deal of my life letting obesity have control over me and finally have found my way to take that control and put it in my hands. I would like to tell you about myself and about parts of my life as I continue with my story. It is my hope that if you relate to anything I have written, that you use it as an opportunity to get to know yourself a little better. I'm not proud of some of the things I will be telling you but if it helps someone else to change, then I feel it is worth sharing.

I am a widowed mother of two. My son is a very accomplished engineering student attending the University of Massachusetts. My daughter is both cognitively and emotionally challenged. She is a very sweet and friendly child, but needs constant care and supervision. My parents, both now deceased, separated when my sister and I were young, and then later divorced. Being raised by a single, working parent is not what most people prefer, but it was better than living in the stressful environment of an unhappy marriage. What does all this have to do with my fight against obesity? It has a lot to do with it because my weight problem was mainly due to my compulsive overeating. I sought out food to be my support and source of comfort, especially through the difficult times in my life. I was looking for a way to cope. Some people turn to food as their crutch and that's what worked for me, or so I thought.

Once I started to hover around the 330-pound mark, I stopped getting on the scale. I didn't want to deal with the reality of my situation. I just kept eating, and the way that I am able to gain weight I know that I probably topped off at around 350 pounds. I didn't start to weigh myself again until I was well into my weight loss program. Within a year, I had cut my weight in half and after seven years I had beat the odds and managed to maintain my weight over the long term. It has been hard work and it gets harder as I get older. My body thinks that it should be obese and that's my fight. There are so many factors working against me that I have little margin for error.

There are times when I would absolutely love to sit down and eat whatever I want. There are times when I hate to go to the gym. Those times don't last long because I know what will happen if I give in. Many people won't survive the test. If there was an easy way out, we would all be the correct weight. Everybody would be lining up for a chance at the magic solution. You have to ask yourself, how much do you want to change and are you willing to turn your back on a lifestyle that isn't good for you?   This is a serious lifetime commitment and it is much better than living with the alternative.

Who is my target audience? It's not going to be fitness-savvy women who already know the things that I want to teach. It is going to be the woman who doesn't know how to take the first step into a better lifestyle. It is going to be the woman who may know the steps but doesn't know how to put them together to make them work for her. It may even be someone who is trying to help another person through a difficult endeavor, but isn't sure how to proceed. Many of us take for granted the knowledge that we have acquired about health and fitness. We assume that in this day and age everybody knows how to lose weight, so what's the problem? The problem is that there are people who don't know how to lose weight and don't know how to keep it off.

I would like you to use what I have written as a handbook or a guide to help you identify what works for you, what works against you and how to find your own source of motivation to develop a plan for success. This book is not just about weight control or whether or not your nail polish should match your lipstick. It is about your well-being and about your outlook on your life. It is about how you feel about yourself and what changes you would like to make. This isn't going to be about becoming a size two or preparing to run a marathon. It is going to be about how you can feel and look your best…whatever that may be for you as an individual. Come to think of it, this can be a type of marathon. Just contemplate all of the great rewards that you could find at the finish line! Picture them in your mind. What changes are you ready for? Change is possible if you possess the right attitude, incentive and will to make the sacrifices to get to where you want to be.

Throughout this book I will take you through various steps that I have found practical and I hope you will find useful in your passage to a new and better you. I don't feel that there is one universal plan of success that is ideal for everyone. Each person's individual needs can be quite diverse or complex, so I may at times offer advice by referring you to a specific source for your information. In this way I feel that I am supplying you with the best combination of material that I can to meet your own needs. I'll tell you about my journey through the eyes of someone who actually lived the life that you may be living right now.

This book may be small, but like a good nutritional plan, it has no fillers or unnecessary additives. It is a straightforward approach of how to rework your thinking as well as your physical condition. By the way, a lot of what I have written can benefit some of the male population too, so if you're so inclined, share and enjoy my little red book together. Gain your own experiences and build on them to write your own story of success.

Part One

Debra L. O'Melia

Building a Foundation for Change

When I tell women my story, I am frequently asked what it was that finally made me want to change. The important thing is that I did have my moment of truth that made me want to do the work on myself and make some positive changes in my life. It doesn't matter what drives me and keeps me motivated, except to me. Everyone is unique and we all have to find that special spark of desire to want something better for ourselves. That moment is different for every woman. Sometimes it's as wonderful as a guardian angel tapping you on the shoulder and leading you in the right direction.

The second question I'm usually asked pertains to how I made those changes I wished for become a reality. How did I do it? What is my secret? When I explain what worked for me I often receive what has become a predictable reaction. I watch expressions quickly change from a look of wide-eyed anticipation to one of obvious disappointment. This happens because I tell them something that most of them already know. I tell them that my changes came about through a lot of self-discipline, perseverance, dedication, and many hours of appropriate and effective courses of physical training. Some of it hasn't been easy and some of it wasn't the way I would have planned it, but it has all been worth it.

I have no magic pill, miracle diet or easy way out. What I would like to show you is a better way out. I would like to present to you a way to succeed that has worked for me and for many other women. Many of us have a certain amount of knowledge about proper nutrition and fitness. The media constantly supplies our society with what experts and amateurs are advocating on the subject of weight control. A good deal of this advice is worthwhile, but some is not. Some of it is unhealthy and some of it is just too good to be true. Most of us know the reality of what will bring about the results that we want. What you need to do now is ask yourself if you are prepared to do the work. If you are ready, good for you! Change can be difficult but it can be spectacular when it generates a positive outcome. Whether you are willing to start making a commitment to yourself or need more time to decide, read on and see what happens.

There may be times when you may not agree with my opinions or points of view. Some of my suggestions may not fit into your plan for success. Those of us who have prevailed know that certain methods do work even though we may not have completely enjoyed them. Many of us come to a point in our lives when we need to have our faces held up to the mirror and take stock in what we want from life. That's what it took for me and that's what it might take for you to make the first move. I want you to know that I have endured some of the same feelings that you may experience while going through your changes. I'm not going to tell you to just grab a carrot stick and a bottle of water and hope for the best. I'm also not going to

4

hand you some blanket solution that is guaranteed to work for the masses but never does anything but fail you in the end. Some of it may not be easy, but it doesn't mean that your efforts have to be unpleasant or boring.

I want you to take a few moments right now to think about yourself. You may not have done that in a while. You have a right to be happy and to feel complete in your world. If someone were to ask you to describe your ideal self-image, what would that be? Are you honestly pleased with how you are, both inside and out? If there are things you don't like, what do you need to do to turn these things around? Give some thought to how you can improve or accentuate the qualities in yourself that you do like.

Sit down and start making a list of your goals. Try to think of the changes that are possible in a short period of time and some you can accomplish over a longer term. Tackling small goals can help fuel your motivation and maintain your interest. It is important to have the proper attitude and to be ready for change. Don't do any of this work just to please other people. You have to want this for yourself. Find a driving force that will make you want to be a winner in all that you do. There is something out there for everyone. You *will* find it, and once you do, grab onto it and don't let go. Will this be a life-changing experience? That's up to you. You must decide the outcome of your story.

Debra L. O'Melia

Conquering Obesity

Obese...it's a term that conjures negative images that the general public has often used against our overweight population. When I started to write this section of the book I was going to title it "Living with Obesity." Then I thought, who wants to live with obesity? People who are obese already know what it's like to live with this problem. Many would not only like to find a way to deal with their situation, but would also like to let others know exactly what it is like to go through life as an obese person. Obese individuals live with the stereotypes every day. They live with the glares, the jokes and the prejudices. The type of treatment that overweight individuals encounter is often permitted and accepted by those who do not understand the causes of obesity or what it is like to live in a world that finds the difficulties of the obese unacceptable. Ridicule and discrimination of the obese are still commonly tolerated in today's "politically correct" society. Even those who do have a problem with their weight are often invited to join in the sarcasm. Have you ever experienced the sinking feeling that came from overlooking an ignorant sneer directed toward you or someone you care about?

As a child I remember watching a friend being taunted on the playground. She was crying uncontrollably from the relentless heckling. I told her to ignore such stupidity but unfortunately, as many of us know that is not always easy to do. I've also experienced the stigma of having an obese parent and having to live through the heartache of watching strangers stare at my mother and judge her merely by her size. I will never forget the time that one of my husband's friends invited us to a Halloween party and asked me if he could borrow a pair of my husband's jeans to wear as a costume. At the time my husband was wearing a size 58/60 waist. Even though I was surprised and very offended by the request, I declined without making my feelings known but I think the expression on my face said enough. I wonder if this person ever stopped to think what it would have been like for his friend to spend an entire evening listening to people laugh at his weight. By the way, this was the same guy who once asked me if "fat people" have sex. I think I responded with: "No, we got our kids out of a cabbage patch!" Great friend, wasn't he?

I know that all the bad experiences that so many of us have had do play a role in how we look at ourselves and how we deal with the ignorance of others. Some of us are relatively new to all this having gained the extra weight as an adult. Others, like me, have spent most of their life dealing with the stigma of obesity. Genetics, medical conditions, poor metabolism, and other factors are valid causes of the condition, but that doesn't mean that we shouldn't try to fight them. Conquering obesity involves more than reducing calories and increasing physical activity. I had to change my thinking about being overweight and why I continued this lifestyle. I know that many obese people say that they are happy with how they are when they are not. They have difficulty admitting that they want to change. Sometimes it's easier to avoid the problem and keep on doing what we know is not good for us. I've been in that place and I don't believe that anyone is satisfied with being obese. I believe that most of these people would like to be released from the daily struggles that come with being excessively overweight. The inability to perform everyday activities comfortably or the frustration that comes from not being able to participate in parts of life that others take for granted should be enough to cause us to stop and evaluate our quality of life.

If you are not satisfied with your circumstances, don't try to convince yourself that you are. Trying to fool yourself into believing everything is fine isn't going to get you where you want to be. You may have someone even more fantastic hiding inside of you longing to show herself. Do the right thing and let her come out. You shouldn't try to conform to society's perfect image but don't be a victim of obesity. Don't be a victim at all! Recognize who you are and your value as a woman. Be comfortable with yourself but don't be complacent. Be happy with how you see yourself and not how others want you to be. Positive change is not about conforming to what the fashion magazines say you should look like. It is about being the best that you can be for yourself. It is about feeling good about yourself, both physically and mentally. None of us need to look like a supermodel, but it would be nice to gracefully slip through a subway turnstile.

Are you are happy and healthy where you are? If you're not, then think about the reasons why. Notice that I said happy *and* healthy. Although I support a person's right to choose the way they live, I need to mention the risk factors associated with carrying too much weight. Heart disease, hypertension, diabetes, added pressure to the bones and joints, and chronic fatigue are just some of the problems that often become part of the package when a person is significantly overweight. It is important to be aware of the special problems that can be created and aggravated by a higher than average weight. We've all heard the excuses defending obesity. Thin people get sick too, I could get hit by a bus tomorrow, etc., etc., etc. Some women may deny it, but many of us would like to make a change for the better. It's *your* choice. You don't have to settle anymore. Don't let obesity have dominion over your life. Obesity isn't your destiny, your bad karma, or your lot in life. You own your body and it should be under your control. If your weight is keeping you from anything that you want to do or that you want to be, then it is time to take command and lead yourself into a new and brighter future.

Overcoming the Obstacles to Success

It's true that we are not all born with the same advantages or raised with the proper guidance. We don't all possess the same skills, financial resources or emotional support in our lives. That shouldn't stop us from seeking out what we need to be successful or exploring the possibilities of success. We all know that success isn't just measured by how much money we have in the bank or by how many toys we own. For some, great achievements may come in the form of financial gain or security. For others it may simply mean doing what they love and enjoying life. Think of the people that you admire that have overcome some of their own obstacles. Their example can provide you with a great source of inspiration in your quest for success. At the same time, think about some of the obstacles that you've already vanquished and use those experiences to help you through other circumstances that you may face.

In 1995, both my mother and my husband died unexpectedly. Within five months, the two most important adults in my life were gone and I felt as though I had been cut loose from a lifeline and was floating without a direction or design for my life. After the death of my husband, I experienced a chain of events that had a negative influence on my life. I tried to keep my husband's business going, but found it very difficult to manage. There were also outside forces working against me, wanting me to fail. I finally sold out to a larger company, but without the revenue generated by the business, I was forced to sell my home in order to avoid foreclosure. I had people pressuring me to resolve my debts, some of them threatening legal action against me. Gradually I managed to get through everything, partially with the assistance of bankruptcy court. I know that this is more information than you probably need to know, but I'm trying to make a point here. A lot of people have gone through these things and more, but have managed to recover and turn their life around. I have to admit that some of this was my own fault. I realize that at times I didn't fight hard enough and I know that part of the reason was that I didn't care enough. I was overwhelmed, depressed, angry and resentful. Everything that I had built with my husband was slipping through my hands and I was letting it happen. I had little interest in saving my ship from sinking. As I had done many times in my life, I purposely put boundaries and limits on myself that kept me from moving forward. I often used my misfortunes as a way to avoid moving on as though they were a safety net against my progress, and I've had to live with the results.

Do you have any obstacles to success? Do you even know if you do or what they are? Have you created some of your own obstacles? Some people fear success because they think it will push them out of their comfort zone. Well maybe it will, but that could often be a good thing. Concentrate on your objectives, and develop your own strategy for success. Be adventurous, try new things, explore your talents and let them flourish. In some ways, I've been afraid of change all my life, even when I wanted changes to happen. Many people hold themselves back because they are afraid of failure. Know your limits, but exceed them whenever possible. Being successful can be scary, but not as much as the possibility of standing still and never moving forward in life. You don't have to settle for a mediocre existence. Old habits can be hard but not impossible to break. Do you traditionally play the role of the perpetual martyr? If so, then end the tradition and begin a new one... one of positive feelings and aspirations. I want you to wince at self-pity. If you like to throw a lot of "pity parties," find something else to do. Many of the people who want to attend are those who are going to help you keep feeling sorry for yourself. It is a waste of time and eventually most people will tire of your lamentations and decline the invitation.

I often waited for the encouragement of others or sought their approval or permission before I considered something new. You can't make everybody happy all of the time. It's impossible, so don't wear yourself out by trying. It's not your responsibility, and you may compromise your own happiness in the process. When we let people take advantage of us or take us for granted, we create another obstacle for ourselves by becoming a victim. I've done that a lot in my life and it has gotten me absolutely nowhere! Don't let others chart your course or tell you that you can't or shouldn't take a chance. Most of us want to be successful in some way, but often don't know how to take the proper steps. You do have to want success to make it happen in a way that will make you happy. Prioritize your life, manage your time wisely and don't procrastinate when chasing your dreams. I've been guilty of not following this advice and have paid a dear price many times in regretful hindsight and missed opportunities. It is important that we learn something from our mistakes and try to prevent making the same ones again and save ourselves the pain of wondering what might have been. I've put off writing this book for far too long. I've spent years encountering articles and listening to talk shows about people who have achieved substantial weight losses telling their stories. I have also witnessed other individuals who have gone through similar obstacles as I, saying the same things that I have wanted to say and giving the same advice that I have wanted to give. That still wasn't enough to persuade me to stop wasting time and get my own message on paper. I now realize that every situation is different and that everyone's story is unique and that my words of encouragement may be just what someone out there needs to hear. Work for what you want. Don't wait for it to be handed to you or depend on others to come through for you. You must oversee your own destiny, from the smallest details to the more important events. If you wait for someone else and trust that they'll do their part to help, you may end up disappointed. You may never get the life of your fantasy, but what are you going to do to improve the life that you have?

Don't use your shortcomings or lack of confidence to create imaginary disabilities. Doing so may needlessly put you at a disadvantage before you even have time to consider your true talents and abilities. I have seen examples of this at the gym. A new member who has never tried any type of aerobic exercise will take one look at the advanced students and immediately declare: "There's no way that I'll ever be able to do that!" They'll give every excuse they can think of to explain away their lack of faith in themselves. I have trained some of these women and my reply is always: "You will do that!" I don't care about the faces that they make back at me. I just go right ahead and show them and then make them try and guess what? Eventually with time and the patience of both them and myself, they find that they can in fact do that and more!

Debra L. O'Melia

Help with Special Problems

When a person begins a weight loss program, it is sometimes not just what they're eating but also what might be eating away at them that can be a stumbling block to their success. Some people hope that weight loss will fix other problems in their life. There may be underlying issues in their life, either past or present, which they have not settled.

Have you ever wanted to sit down and have an open and honest conversation with someone about your life? A casual chat with a friend or a heartfelt dialogue with a loved one can be helpful, but do you feel that you need more? There may come a time when you need to speak to someone who doesn't have any emotional ties to you and who can be more objective about your situation. You may not even realize the full scope of what is troubling you without the aid of someone who is trained to help you sort out your problems in the proper way.

Some people may feel helpless or alone in the world. Still others may be battling some form of addiction or multiple addictions and feeling out of control and unable to cope with the hold that their compulsions have on them. Many women are in a troubled or harmful relationship and don't know how to change their situation. Some people worry excessively or feel very anxious or nervous or have difficulty dealing with change or loss.

If you can identify with these or any other critical issues that are threatening your well-being or even your own survival, you need to seek out someone who can help you make sense of it all and can work with you in finding a solution. You deserve the proper care and attention. I cannot emphasize enough the importance of addressing this part of your plan. It may be a vital component and may very well be the cornerstone in building a new and better life.

Your physician can assist you by evaluating your condition, making a diagnosis or referring you to a colleague who specializes in your particular needs. Like a good support group, you may have to look for the provider that makes you feel comfortable and understands the matters you wish to resolve. Don't be afraid to ask for help and don't be shy about asking for credentials from those in which you would place your trust. However, you must also play an active role in your care. You should be straightforward and sincere and be a willing and cooperative patient. A good flow of communication between you and your doctor or therapist is very important for a successful treatment plan.

Although I've learned to fight a lot of my own battles, I've also learned how to ask for help when I need it. I've been helped by some very special people in my life, from friends to professionals. Some have been more of an influence than others, but each one of them has added something to who I am today. Sometimes you already know certain things about yourself need to change, but you need someone else to push you into doing something about it. I've had to study some harsh realities about myself but it has made me someone who I like better than the person I was before. I've had to look at myself in ways that weren't always attractive but coming out of denial about oneself can be a very healing experience.

If you are apprehensive or fearful, seek out a companion to stand by you. It might be your significant other, a relative, trusted friend, or religious advisor. If you prefer to remain anonymous, there are health facilities such as your local hospital or clinic that can guide you in the right direction. In any event, it is important to remember that if you need help make it a top priority to get that help. Your mental health and self-esteem are every bit as important a part in all of this as is your physical health and fitness. Don't forfeit the chance to finally break the chains that may be holding you back from being all you long to be. Take that first step and know that it will very likely be one of the most significantly good things that you will ever do for yourself.

Debra L. O'Melia

Knowing Your Saboteurs

An important lesson that many women need to learn is how to be true to themselves and to eliminate antagonistic influences from their lives. Too many of us put ourselves on the back burner and frequently lose sight of what we genuinely desire and what will make us happy. We are often so preoccupied with taking care of business and trying to please others that our own needs get pushed aside. Don't try to fit in to an image of what someone else wants you to be. Our goals and achievements are ultimately our own responsibility, but people that are feeding you their negative attitudes or are being unresponsive to your changes are not contributing to your progress. They may help to discourage your efforts. Don't allow others to block your path to fulfillment.

Before I began a fitness plan, I already had people in my life that helped to reinforce my poorly chosen lifestyle. You may have some of them in your life. The relatives who told you, "You have such a pretty face, don't worry about the rest." The friend from high school who laments, "I don't know why you're so interested in all this self-improvement stuff anyway. I don't care what *I* look like!" or one of my personal favorites: "Hey, life is short, so just enjoy yourself!" Great philosophy at work there! Some of the most common carriers of sabotage are the helpful individuals who will try to talk you into breaking training by feeling sorry for you and your endeavor to lose weight. They may try to help you out with a statement like: "Oh, come on! You've been so good, you deserve to treat yourself!" This statement can open up the door to temptation and you then have to decide whether or not to walk through and live with the consequences. Think about this for a moment: If you were a recovering alcoholic, would your friends come up to you and say, "Hey, you've been sober for six months! Come on, have a drink! You deserve it!"? It's wonderful to hear an encouraging voice say, "You've done so well, don't spoil all your hard work. It's not worth it." That's the kind of friend you should be listening to. Remember that the same people who cheered you on to indulge are probably not going to be there the next day to help you work off what you may have gained by giving in to their provocation. Once you do start progressing into your program, these may be the same people that will offer you the least amount of encouragement. You need to be aware of these opposing influences because they are what may affect your confidence in your ability to carry out your program. Unsupportive people are sometimes jealous of the accomplishments of others because they may be insecure about something in their own life. You may find many people that will be very proud of you and will offer you lots of reinforcement. That kind of backing is very important, especially in those times when you are feeling a little doubtful about your progress.

It's good to have a support network. If you don't, then you may have to go out and find one. Try a support group that specializes in weight control and eating difficulties. You may already be familiar with some organizations. They can often be found in the phone book, on the internet, or through public service agencies or health care providers. There are some very good and well-established groups that have helped many women and they could very well provide you with an excellent source of stability when you need it the most. You may need to do a little research to find the place where you will feel most comfortable. If you're not interested in joining a group but still feel that you need a little push in the right direction, ask a friend who is interested in self-improvement to be your fitness partner and work together.

Some of your saboteurs may be right under the same roof with you. This can create some difficulty because it is almost impossible to avoid their poor frame of mind. (Notice that I said *almost* impossible.) Support on the home front is very important, and you should try to cultivate some cooperation there. Chances are you are not the only one in the house that is in need of a little modification.

Don't be your own worst enemy. You may set yourself up for failure if you hold others responsible for something that you can and should control. I've had women tell me things like, "I'm really upset with my husband! Last night he brought home all of this junk food so, of course, I just *had* to eat some too!" Don't blame your husband, your mother, your kids or anyone else for your lack of conviction. Using scapegoats and making excuses for your own mistakes is a waste of time. What you should be doing is concentrating on yourself and how you want all of this to turn out for you. I know that you are setting out to do something that can be very difficult and frustrating. You need to recognize your weak points and protect yourself from things that will invite you to fail. Learn to identify the danger signals and when you need to run for help. Always remember to stay strong and keep your goals in sight!

Part Two

Debra L. O'Melia

Redesigning Yourself

Plus size, queen size, full figured. Whatever is the popular term at the time is what we are labeled. What qualifies a woman to be "plus-sized?" I remember when it meant anyone size 14/16 and over. Often now even a size 10/12 is considered the minimum. What's next, size 6/8? It's no wonder so many women and young girls are risking their health trying to fit into the mold of what others dictate is the ideal.

I know that there are many plus women that are fulfilled and aware of their gifts and talents and may not need any advice on physical self-improvement. It's great when a woman knows she is beautiful, well adjusted and happy with her life. Some of us need a little help and direction to get us to that special place. Today's plus woman should be healthy and fit. The times are changing and the conventional image of a full-figured woman as being matronly and unattractive is being shattered by confident, sexy and vibrant ladies all over the world. We have curves, and that's great! Let's not hide them under excess pounds that we know we don't need. Even plus-sized models are encouraged to firm, tone and adjust their weight to produce a more sculpted look for the camera. We can be realistically proportioned but still continue to improve and restyle ourselves.

Once you have established a better understanding of how to change your thinking about obesity, it should be easier to approach the actual work involved. Think about how much weight you want to lose and how you would like to accomplish your task. Proper diet and exercise are a great team. Together they help us to get the job done more efficiently. Your fitness plan, program, regime or whatever you choose to call it must be tailored especially for you. In this section of the book I will show you how to personalize your method of weight loss to get the best results for you as an individual. Not every plan works the same way for every woman. It is very important to find the right formula to insure your own personal success.

Getting Started

Before you begin, it may be a good idea to get your physician's approval before you consider any new fitness plan. This is particularly important if you have any specific medical conditions or are taking any special medications. If it has been a while since your last physical, make an appointment for a checkup. Let your doctor know your intentions and see if there will be any restrictions on diet or exercise. Yes, do request permission to exercise. Ask your doctor his or her opinion on what would be a safe amount and what types of fitness activities you could tolerate. Ask for their help in mapping out a fitness blueprint that will work for you. Choose one that you can stick to on a long term basis and that can be easily made more challenging as your endurance improves. Your physician may also refer you to the services of a registered dietician or certified personal trainer for additional guidelines. Please take advantage of their experience. Individual counseling can be very helpful and effective, especially when you are unsure of how to proceed with a weight control program.

When you have a substantial weight loss goal in mind, it may sometimes seem like an overwhelming mission because of the time and effort that will be required to reach your destination. This can sometimes be discouraging for many women and can often lead to a feeling of defeat before even giving themselves a chance. Don't try to take on too much all at once. If you're feeling uneasy about your new challenge, avoid giving complete attention to the total scope of your plan at first. Try to break up your goals into smaller, manageable segments. This is a more sensible approach and helps to increase the possibility of your success. Holidays and special occasions served as great milestones on which to chart my weight loss timetable. I would pick a holiday and use that as a target date for the next goal that I wanted to achieve. Be realistic and sensible. Don't set your expectations so high that you give yourself too little a margin of time to achieve satisfying results. Trying to lose weight too quickly in too small an amount of time is not only difficult, but doing so may compromise your health as well.

Your physician can suggest a safe standard of weight loss for you to follow based on your physical condition. Keep your doctor informed of your progress so that they can evaluate your health status. The scale can be your friend or foe. It can be a good monitor of your progress, but if it is constantly beckoning to you to hop on, forget it. Don't walk a tightrope every day with the numbers. There are factors that can make a woman's weight rise unexpectedly which can lead to frustration when chasing your goal. Weighing yourself once a week should be sufficient. Instead of obsessing about the scale, pay attention to how you are feeling, how your clothes are fitting, and even how your energy level may be improving.

Several factors may influence the efficiency of your weight program, the most apparent being your total caloric intake and the extent of your physical activity. Exercise (yes, I said exercise again), in any reasonable amount will assist in speeding up the whole process. How efficiently the body's metabolism functions varies from one person to another and is what helps to decide how you burn away your "extra you." In the beginning of your program you may find that you are experiencing very steady and productive results and that after a period of time you start to level off. These weight plateaus are normal and are usually only temporary delays. You should never allow them to dampen your spirit or use them as a reason to give up. This might not be easy, but give it a chance. More importantly, give yourself a chance! Whatever problems you do have with losing weight can usually be overcome in some way. Don't worry about the big picture. Start with baby steps and take little snapshots of yourself along the way.

Debra L. O'Melia

Establishing a Healthy Relationship with

Food

For most of my life my relationship with food has not been a very good one. I know that some people joke about being born hungry, but in my case it was actually true. My mother had, as the story goes, experienced a difficult and prolonged labor. She had not been feeling well and had eaten almost nothing in three days. When I finally did arrive, I was born with ten little chewed fingertips. The doctor said that I had tried to compensate for my lack of sustenance by nibbling on my fingers. Well, I think that I spent the next four decades making up for those three days!

Growing up in the sixties, I remembered there was always somewhere for me to perfect the art of passionate food enjoyment. Fast food establishments, theaters, ice cream stands, and anything else that could attract the new growing population of young families were rapidly increasing in numbers. Television's popularity created a whole new dimension in temptation with all those inviting commercials in "living color." It was the beginning of TV's contribution to our increasingly sedentary lifestyle.

Family picnics and other food-related activities were as popular as ever. There were also the holidays to look forward to as well. They provided us with our own free pass to "pig-out" heaven!

Speaking of pigs (No, I'm not going to insult anyone), my family would often patronize a local creamery whose specialty of the house was a decadent dessert called a "pig's dinner." This simple little treat basically consisted of about six scoops of ice cream, three bananas, hot fudge, both pineapple and strawberry sauces, whipped cream, nuts and, of course, the traditional cherry on top. All this was served up in what looked like some sort of paper bucket that would have either challenged or disgusted anyone but the most seasoned connoisseur of this type of sweet creation. Sounds incredible, doesn't it? What's incredible is that even at the age of eight, I was more than able to devour an entire "dinner" of my very own with no effort whatsoever!

A lot of baby boomers found themselves in the post-war land of plenty when it came to food. No sir, no one was ever going to go hungry again! It was "Clean your plate, there are starving children in the world." Well, looking back, I think that we should have fed our children less and sent a check to a worthy charity to help feed those hungry children. Our fat cells were developing quite nicely with our parents often oversupplying our diets during the week and well-meaning Depression Era grandparents taking up the slack on the weekends with their own ethnic means of subversion. I was blessed with two grandmothers who loved to eat and got great pleasure out of watching me do the same. My maternal grandmother was Polish and my paternal grandmother was Portuguese. The two of them kept me well supplied with all of their specialties and I never disappointed them with my enjoyment of their efforts. A good deal of my generation was now unknowingly beginning our life-long, love-hate relationship with food.

In the early seventies I met my future husband who had also inherited a passion for food. What fun we had feasting and "growing" together! By the time our son and daughter came along in the eighties, I was well on my way to my top weight of over three hundred pounds. I didn't need to buy maternity clothes. I simply kept on wearing my everyday tent dresses and elastic waist pants. My capacity for food was nothing short of astonishing. I could now consume more food than anyone I knew, including my own husband. My daily menu was chocked full of doughnuts, bagels, pasta, sandwiches, ice cream or whatever else was on hand. I would never have any difficulty stuffing down three huge meals every day and after putting the kids to bed, I would join my husband in front of the TV for a "snack." I could easily make a whole package of cookies or an entire half-gallon of ice cream disappear in one sitting.

Although the early nineties brought many changes to my life, my poor eating habits remained intact. Instead of evaluating my situation and putting my life on a more constructive course, I plunged myself even deeper into the trough of apathy that I had dug for myself. I enjoyed self-pity almost as much as my beloved ice cream and wallowed in both of them on a regular basis. It was easier for me to reach for something to eat than it was to reach out for a better life. I had convinced myself that this was the way I would spend the rest of my life. I isolated myself from the world and insulated myself from my problems with the help of my most loyal companion… food.

Do you have a bond with food? Is it an unhealthy relationship? Has it brought you superficial gratification but let you down and left you with feelings of guilt and regret? Maybe it's time to rethink this coupling of yours and see what you can do to turn the tide in this unhappy union. What does food do for you? The benefits of sound nutritional habits are long lasting, but the good feelings that the act of eating may provide are fleeting. Does food make you happy? Does it solve your problems? Does it fill a need that should be satisfied by something else in your life? It may be time for you to examine the importance that you give food in your life. Maybe it's not as good a friend as you thought. It's possible that you've been giving it too much credit and spending too much time nurturing this one-sided affair. Perhaps you should be putting more of your energy into something more worthwhile that will provide you with real and enduring satisfaction.

You may sometimes hear women say: "I don't know why I have so much trouble losing weight. I really don't eat that much." Maybe they don't or maybe they're not eating the right foods or have no set eating schedule. The truth is that so many of us eat the wrong foods and combine them with too much inactivity that we are giving our bodies a great lesson in Fat Storage 101! If you feel that you may be overeating, think of your body as an overstocked refrigerator. You now need to take inventory and use up some of the food stores you already have. Supply your body with the necessities to keep it adequately nourished and don't add excess provisions. In other words, start cutting back on the junk while you continue a steady supply of healthy foods in your diet.

When you eat, is it always because you are actually hungry, or do you often find yourself eating purely for the diversion that it provides? Have you ever asked yourself, "Why am I eating this?" Do you ever find that you don't even want to eat but you eat just because the food is there? Do you often eat well beyond the point that your hunger has been satisfied? Perhaps you find eating is a gratifying way to pass the time like it's some sort of sporting event (only this activity will add calories, not burn them). Some of the biggest culprits that lead us into this pattern of "recreational eating" include watching television, talking on the phone, boredom, depression, and of course, social occasions where this kind of eating is always encouraged. Try to find something else to do during certain activities or moods to turn your attention away from food. If you stick with it, over time you will eventually learn the difference between a craving and real hunger. Sometimes when you feel a craving all it might be is your body telling you it needs a drink, not a pastrami and cheese sandwich. It may surprise you that a glass of water or a hot cup of tea may be just enough to quiet those hunger pangs. Don't go to a party or other event hungry. Eat something that is on your plan before you go to prevent you from devouring everything in sight upon your arrival. A partially full stomach will help to intercept you from eating too much.

Remember, you're there for the fun and good company, not to see how much food you can gulp down!

Avoid eating late at night, preferably not after eight o'clock. Your body is more prone to store what you have eaten, and it will be that much harder to burn the calories effectively. If you're not a morning person, rediscover breakfast. The importance of this meal is not underestimated. It jumpstarts your body and provides you with a good nutritional foundation for the rest of the day. Knowing this, you will certainly make good menu choices, won't you? (A slice of last night's pizza and two jelly doughnuts does not qualify!) Once you delete your nighttime munching, you'll be surprised at how much of a welcome treat breakfast can be. Never skip meals. You're not doing yourself a favor by starving all day. Depriving your body of enough food is like an insurance policy against successful weight loss. You may even interfere with your metabolism because your body will go into a panic mode at the threat of starvation and will actually refuse to cooperate with your attempts to lose weight. Your body does mean well. It is not trying to make your life miserable, but it has a job to do and will fight to protect itself. Never be too busy to eat well. Take the time and it will pay great dividends in the long run.

Try to break up your food consumption into several small meals throughout the day. This helps to control your hunger, and can also create a steadier metabolism. If you're like an Olympic sprinter with a fork, learn to eat slowly and remember to put your implement of destruction down between bites. These practices do help to make you feel full sooner and prevent you from overdoing at mealtime. Relax; the food isn't going to jump off your plate. For all you gold medal eaters that like to inhale your meal, put the plate down and stop shoveling! My husband used to make vacuum cleaner noises while he watched me eat. Sometimes he would look at me in amazement and say: "Calm down, Deb! Don't scrape the pattern off the plate." He would also occasionally remind me that the plate itself was indeed not edible.

Don't eat while cooking, and avoid the temptation to sample. You're only racking up a whole bunch of calories before you even sit down at the table. Try keeping a glass of ice water or some other calorie free beverage nearby to sip on. This will not only keep your mouth busy, but it will also help to subdue those pre-dinner urges. If you need to chew something, try a salad, some raw vegetables, or some sugarless gum. I know that none of these things may be what you really want, but they're better than high-calorie alternatives.

Try eating in front of a mirror. Getting "up close and personal" while stuffing your face can be a real eye opener and bring you into reality about how you eat. Observe each and every bite. Do you hunch over your plate like starving wildlife? Do you covet that bag of potato chips or cookies like it is the last one you'll ever find? If you don't like what you see, then do something about it. Guilt can be a great appetite suppressant and a great motivator.

We all know that improving our eating habits will involve some lifestyle changes. It is important to acquire the proper attitude toward food. Many of us have walked down this path and now it is time to find the right direction, and that may take a while. The "one day at a time" rule may apply here, especially if you are trying to change for the first time or if you have a long road to travel. If you have to take it one hour at a time, then do so. Take whatever time you need to make things work in your favor. You need to get to a point in your life where how you feel and how you look mean more to you than your enjoyment of food.

Dealing with Compulsive Overeating

Food... we need it to stay alive, but many of us have trouble living *with* it. Unlike other things that are addictive, food cannot be omitted from our daily routine. It is sometimes difficult for outsiders to understand this problem. They argue that it should be easier for overeaters because they still get to eat, they just have to learn to control themselves. People that are addicted to food know that restraining their obsession is not an easy task. What would it be like for an alcoholic to keep drinking in limited amounts, or a heavy smoker to live with a very controlled number of cigarettes? When people look at it in this way, it may be easier for them to realize the unique situation of the food addict. Compulsive overeaters who want to change their habits need to handle their preoccupation with food by creating a delicate balance between moderation and an all-encompassing desire.

Another common misconception among those who don't understand this eating disorder is that not all obese individuals are compulsive overeaters. The image of an overweight person as being one who is constantly binging on excess amounts of food is a depiction that is formed by opinions that are uneducated and judgmental. Obesity may be a result of compulsive overeating, but the two do not always go hand in hand. The uncontrollable urge to overeat is a complex problem that needs to be addressed with a measure of tolerance and sensitivity. If you need help, let your feelings be known and stop swallowing them along with all of the food.

Eating had, for most of my life, been my favorite pastime. Most of the time it was my only one. Food was my friend and my comfort and I surrounded myself with others who felt the same way. After all, what fun were people who didn't enjoy the sheer pleasure of overindulgence? To me, eating was so much fun (at least my idea of fun), that I really didn't care about what I was doing to myself. In reality, I was already setting myself up for a lifetime struggle with food. It took me years to face the fact that I was a compulsive overeater. My compulsion was so severe that my drive to consume large amounts of food ruled over me each and every day.

My appetite was insatiable. Even when I was in the middle of a meal, I would anticipate its end with disappointment and frustration. I would eat during meal preparation, between meals, and soon after a meal was finished I would resume my fanatical behavior without giving much thought to the consequences. If I attended a social function where food was served, I would be overcome with both a feeling of anticipation and one of anxiety. I was overjoyed that I was surrounded by food, but at the same time I was actually worried that there wouldn't be enough for me. I remember trying to figure out how I would get to sample something from each item before others had the audacity to help themselves and leave none for me! "All you can eat" gatherings are heaven on earth to a compulsive overeater, but are as bad an idea for them as an open bar is to a person with a drinking problem. Most people do enjoy good food in moderation, but compulsives go too far and cross the line into obsession. They don't have the luxury of using food for simple enjoyment or as an enhancement to social interaction. To do so only gets them into trouble by taunting their lack of self-control.

If you are in a battle with food, then you must learn to turn it from being your nemesis to what it was originally intended to be, which is a source of nutrition and fortification. You need to gather your arsenal of defense and develop a strategy to bring about your victory over food and eventually call a truce and make peace with your adversary. How do you do that? A good way is to evaluate the impact that food has on your life. I'm not talking about the sustenance that it provides, but about the dependency that you may have on it and how its use affects your daily living.

You need to think of food as fuel. I'm not saying that eating should never be a pleasant experience. Good food should be enjoyed. Wonderful aromas, colors, tastes and textures are what make food appealing and satisfying. However, food should not be a substitute for something else, like love or emotional support. Those needs should be met in other ways. Eating should not be used as a psychological crutch or as a way to escape from problems. Food is an inanimate object. It doesn't love, nurture or provide guidance. It can't be your friend and it never has been. Getting a pet or finding an interesting hobby is a better source of comfort and happiness than food will ever be and you must try to find replacements for food in certain aspects of your of life. What are *you* hungry for? Is it food or is it something else?

Do you eat to live or do you live to eat? Does overeating have such a hold on you that it controls and dictates how you will spend your day? Have you even admitted to yourself that you have a real problem with food? Compulsive overeating goes beyond satisfying simple cravings or occasionally giving in to boredom or mood swings. Food addicts are plagued with a constant need to pursue the object of their fixation. People with this problem need to explore the reasons why they eat this way and find a solution. They need to find something that will take away their hunger. Something that they will love more than food.

I had to realize what I was doing to myself, both physically and emotionally. I know how much a compulsive wants to eat, and I know how much they want to stop eating. Over the years, I have tried to find my own ways to break this behavior pattern. Some are as simple as walking away from temptation or as profound as looking inside myself to understand why I was eating and what I was really looking for in my life. This change didn't happen in a short period of time but it's a wonderful feeling to finally be in a place where I have the control I need to keep myself from falling back into my past. Do your best to find your place as well. Want this to happen with all your heart and know that it is possible. Anything is if you truly believe.

Living with Sensible Nutrition

Now that you have a good base of information about how you should eat, let's do a little research about what you should be eating. Many people who grew up in the same era as I did (that is, the days before reading nutritional labels and getting the proper amounts of exercise) found it very easy to eat themselves into a state of "morbid obesity." (I would like to know who invented that particular description.) Excess consumption of fat, salt, and sugar were not even given a second thought. Many of us went through the trials of the latest fad diets and soon found out how ineffective they were. My family's health history read like a medical version of a horror novel full of victims of heart disease and diabetes, but that did not stop me from taxing my system with all sorts of evil delicacies.

First of all, forget the idea of diet and deprivation. One of the reasons diets fail is that they often restrict us to the point where we are too hungry and frustrated to follow through for any length of time. Did you ever notice that you feel more tempted to overeat when you are on a strict diet than when you're not? Our bodies not only need the proper types of fuel, but also the right amounts, to keep everything in the best condition for successful weight loss and maintenance. I have come to the conclusion, as many other life-long dieters have, that many methods of weight loss are impractical and usually lead to unrealistic expectations. Many of them lead us right into failure and do not teach us how to sustain satisfactory results. Good luck with the latest miracle diet of the week! If they are such miracles, then why are so many of us excessively overweight? If you think that fad diets are going to bring you lasting results, you're probably in for a big surprise. Although you may experience positive results initially, these results may be extremely difficult or impossible to maintain.

Educate yourself and get ready to rework your nutritional lifestyle. Choose a well-balanced nutritional plan that will work for you. Remember that feeling you would get on the first day of a new diet? That sinking feeling that came with the realization that for what seemed like the next hundred years you would be sentenced to a menu of grapefruit, black coffee, and dried toast? If you were really good, you could always reward yourself with a cup of diet gelatin (*yum!*). Hey, we've all tried the two ounces of tuna on a lettuce leaf. Let's eat something that will make us want to stick to healthy eating habits. In some respects many of us are diet experts. We all know little tricks of the trade from years of trying different diets and from comparing notes with others who have gone through the same trials of weight loss. Unfortunately, many of us still haven't found the right formula to work for us.

Eat a well-balanced diet, and if you have any doubts about what that may mean for you, please consult your doctor or seek the advice of a registered dietician or other nutrition expert to help sort things out. Some are available for a small fee or may be covered by your insurance. Check with your local hospital to see if they offer free nutritional services. Many people have individual nutritional needs that may be dictated by age, medical conditions, or other factors. In such cases, special dietary guidelines may apply. It is important to find the right mix of nutrients, portion sizes, and meal planning to help insure your best rate of healthy weight loss.

What works for one woman may not work for another. Consulting with a nutrition counselor is a good way to find out what you may need to change about your diet. You may be eating too much of one food group and not enough of another. Certain foods may be helping to slow your progress or you may be eating something that may be overstimulating your appetite. Getting an overview of your eating habits through the use of a dietary journal is also useful in planning an effective nutritional regimen.

Always take the time to refuel, no matter how busy you are. That doesn't mean stopping for a quick snack of pastry or French fries. It may not seem like much at the time, but those nasty little calories are always adding up. Little things do mean a lot. Just because you ate a small handful of junk food instead of a healthy meal, don't think you're winning the game. Read the nutritional label on all your favorite treats while you contemplate how long they will fill your hunger gap between meals. *Now* how do they taste?

I didn't find it necessary to purchase any specially prepared foods. In my opinion, food is food. You can use it to your advantage naturally and simply to get the results you want. Avoid excess sugar and salt. Watch your servings of bread, crackers, pasta and refined sugars. Try to choose fish and poultry over red meat, and stay away from processed foods and deli meats. Vegetables are a good source of vitamins and fiber and can help calm the urge to eat by filling your stomach. Choose fresh or frozen rather than canned to cut down on sodium. Limit starchy vegetables like corn and peas. If you don't already include them in your diet, try to acquire a taste for skim milk, fat-free sliced or cottage cheese and yogurt over the high-fat alternatives. Eat whole fresh fruits rather than drinking a lot of juice to get the greatest nutritional benefit. Limit consumption of high-sugar fruits such as grapes and tropical fruits.

Most fast food chains have finally realized that there is a market for healthy food choices. Be aware of what they have to offer and utilize this convenient way of staying on your plan. Once you become accustomed to this way of eating, you should be able to establish a regular dietary routine. You should feel better, look better and improve your chance for a healthier life.

"To Cheat or Not to Cheat"

Cheating on a weight loss plan can be like playing a game of chance. Unless you are very confident in your ability to maintain adequate self-control, it is best that you don't set out on a cheating adventure. This can be especially important to consider if you are in the early stages of your quest to change your eating habits. Cheating is a skill that many women have to learn over time as they get to know their own powers of restraint. When you do have cravings it is essential that you master a control over your urges and manage them right from the start. It is possible to find a suitable balance between self-indulgence and deprivation. It's important to learn how to cheat in a worthwhile manner that will leave you satisfied but will not disrupt your fitness plan.

If you find yourself yearning for something, don't deprive yourself. However, before you give in to your craving, I want you to observe these specific rules of the cheating game. Make sure that you absolutely must possess this immediate gratification. Ask yourself some critical questions: Is this something that I simply cannot get through the next few minutes or hours without, or could I possibly find something else to shift my attention to until the urge passes? If I do give in, will I be able to stop myself or will this little indiscretion ignite my appetite and cause me to suffer a binge attack? Will I feel guilty when the fun is over, and how much of my progress will it have cost me? Is it worth jeopardizing my progress? It may seem like I'm making a big deal about something that should be simple, but I want you to understand how important all this could be in you program.

Once you have cheated, this does not give you permission to go on an eating spree. Don't try to convince yourself that you "blew it," and therefore you might as well start all over again tomorrow, or on Monday, after the holidays, or whenever the spirit moves you. Get right back on track and resume your plan immediately, before you feel that you are at the point of no return. You made a conscious choice to indulge. It's over; deal with it, and move on.

Now if after all your soul searching, you do finally come to the conclusion that you simply can no longer resist temptation, you should cheat with the item that you really want and use no substitutes. If you are dreaming of that fantastic chocolate cake from the bakery down the street, then that is what you should pursue. If the bakery is closed, you can wait until the next day; you'll survive. Maybe by then you'll have already conquered your craving and saved yourself a whole bunch of empty calories! The reason why I am advocating this *all or nothing* approach is that if you don't have exactly what you want you may very well end up eating your way through a whole trail of other food that you don't really want because your original craving was never satisfied. If your favorite bakery is closed and you are in a crisis situation, by all means do seek out another chocolate cake. Just make sure that it as close as possible in quality to your true heart's desire to insure your complete contentment.

Before you plunge into that chocolate cake, French vanilla ice cream, or freshly baked bread, please understand that you can't give yourself permission to consume the entire cake or whole container of ice cream or loaf of bread. Know your limits. Once you have picked your "poison," you may only enjoy one portion (one *reasonable* portion, that is), and no more! Eventually with practice and some self-control, you will train your body and your psyche to be comfortable with just enough of your treat to see you through your period of longing. Don't bring home three cakes or two gallons of ice cream. It doesn't matter if it was hard to find, on sale or free! Don't bring it home. Many of your bad eating habits will occur at home where your supply of forbidden goodies is often most available. You need to cheat-proof your environment as much as possible and the best way to do so is to eliminate the dangerous articles in the first place.

Use your common sense and make careful choices, ultimately trying to get as close to the real thing as possible to help guarantee a quick and painless break in your fitness plan. Don't cheat with additional items that are not on your original menu of delight. Stay faithful to the idea of a single item and include nothing extra. Don't decide that you'll have some of that incredible gourmet ice cream on the side with your chocolate cake or maybe lead into your glorious dessert with a fabulously rich main course. Forget about it! Don't get carried away, especially if you are still unsophisticated at playing this little game.

Never use food as a reward. Your cheat should be used to satisfy a craving and not to pat you on the back for losing five pounds. If you had quit smoking for a month, would you compensate yourself by lighting up? There are plenty of other ways to give yourself a round of applause. I'm sure that you can think of plenty all on your own. Finding alternative reward methods may also keep your mind off of food. Give yourself some time. Your chance will come to advance into the world of culinary pleasures. Try to be patient; I think you will find that it is definitely worth the wait!

Effective Maintenance Techniques

Preserve your achievements and never stop improving, changing or succeeding. Always remain a work in progress. When you do reach your goal lock the door on any chance to return to your old way of life. Take your success, run with it and don't look back. As your fitness program moves forward you need to remain aware of how far you have traveled and what you need to do to stay on the right path. Many women become overly confident with their new command over their weight. Many of us have a body that has been so programmed over the years to retain large amounts of weight that it is very difficult to get the old information to "leave the terminal." Some of that information will always be ready to rear its ugly head whenever we provide it the opportunity.

There may even come a time when you will serve as a role model for someone else. People may treat you differently and also lavish you with praise for what you have done. Some might even look to you for advice and guidance. That's a lot to live up to. People around you may even start to monitor your weight, watch what you eat, and check to see if you are being faithful to your fitness program. It doesn't matter how much weight they may have gained or whether or not they are exercising. They will put the spotlight on you. How convenient for them! Having these watchdogs can be a good thing because it could make you feel honor bound to forever maintain your final results. Their interest in you could help you stay focused on yourself. Their constant attention may even make you feel a little guilty when you gain a few pounds or skip too many days of exercise. It doesn't matter that those who have decided to oversee your progress may not have been doing anything to improve themselves, but they insist on checking what you're up to. This type of supervision can either be amusing or annoying, but it has certainly proven to be one of my best sources of motivation. Always remember that you should be doing this for yourself and not to please someone else.

A very important way to promote effective maintenance is to rid yourself of what we women like to call our "fat" clothes. Give them away, sell them, throw them out. It doesn't matter how you do it, just remove them from your life forever! Many of us find it too easy to eat our way right back into them size by size. This rule not only applies to what you were wearing at your top weight, but also includes whatever clothing you needed to acquire on your way to your goal weight. If you find yourself faltering a bit and your clothes start to feel a little tight, that's your warning signal to get back on track. Having nothing to wear will be a good incentive, don't you think? Remember to use the fit of your clothing as a useful gauge of your weight control. Don't think about going up even one size. The moment that you do you are giving yourself permission to enter dangerous territory that you know you don't ever want to revisit. If you feel that you need some type of memento to remind you of your past transgressions, keep a few "before" photos. Put them up on the refrigerator, bathroom mirror, in your car or anywhere they can haunt you and bring you back to reality when you need to fight temptation. Place one or two of your "worst ever" shots into your purse or gym bag, and be proud to show them off. Seeing the reactions of others and hearing their praises of your accomplishments is a great morale booster and reinforces your commitment.

Maintain a healthy diet and continue to make the right choices. Don't isolate yourself at mealtimes. Sit down with family or friends and enjoy a satisfying dinner. You don't have to feel bad about eating something delicious. Use your common sense and what you have learned about managing your self-control. As you become more experienced in how to stabilize your fitness plan you will become more comfortable with each type of situation involving food and how to adjust your eating habits. Over time you should be able to introduce formerly forbidden foods into your diet and enjoy them in moderation. When dining out, ask the restaurant to make modifications to your order to make it fit into your nutrition plan. Try to remember that you are there for the company, the atmosphere, or just some quiet time alone with your thoughts. It's great to savor a good meal, but you are not there to gorge yourself. Concentrate on your surroundings, not what's on your plate.

Don't neglect your exercise program. Keep moving and remind your body and your metabolism who's in charge. Exercise is an important tool to keep your appetite at bay and one of your best defenses against a weight gain relapse. The added benefits of a regular fitness schedule, such as increased energy and motivation will help to maintain a good attitude toward continued success and remind you why you did all of this in the first place. Never lose sight of what you have now realized and what it took to get yourself there.

Developing the Proper Approach to

Exercise

Many women have found that if anything comes close to a silver bullet regarding weight loss and control, exercise is it. What is your definition of exercise? Fitness experts do not consider carpooling the kids all over town or running errands a suitable exercise program. Cardiovascular fitness is essential to good health and an appropriate exercise program can provide a multitude of benefits including a more efficient metabolism, better sleeping patterns, relief of stress and an improvement in your overall emotional well-being. It is important to include adequate amounts of exercise in your fitness regime. Think of exercise as one of your biggest health and beauty investments.

I hated gym class when I was in school and was not interested in exercise for most of my life. The thought of having to participate in any organized program of physical activity sent me into a frenzied panic, and I gave myself no opportunity to burn any more calories than was absolutely necessary. I thought fitness enthusiasts were obsessed and at times a little obnoxious. I didn't realize at the time how ignorant I was to the world of exercise and that I could have learned something from these "fanatics." About twenty years ago, I decided to join a gym for the first time. The size two spandex goddess sitting behind the front desk looked up at me, all wide-eyed and proudly declared, "Oh, I know just how you feel... I used to be a size twelve!" A size twelve?! Well, I knew right then and there that this woman would never be able to relate to my problems with my weight.

However, in defense of all the size twos of the world, I now know, after years of enlightening conversations with weight battlers of all sizes, we all have some things in common. One woman's own personal struggle might seem insignificant to another, but each is important in its own right. It took me many years to actually be open minded enough to sympathize with rather than resent a 115 pound woman when she complained about how uncomfortable she felt because she had gained five pounds. To her this was a real problem in need of a real solution.

How you perceive the importance of exercise in your life will effect your ability to open up to the possibility of joining the ranks of the physically fit. Maybe you have had some bad experiences and have been turned off to the idea that exercise can actually be fun and quite rewarding. Perhaps you are self-conscious and don't feel confident enough to participate at a public facility. In that case, I recommend an all women's fitness center, where you may be more comfortable and less intimidated than you might be at a co-ed gym. I'm not trying to push a gym membership on you, but it has been my experience that many individuals do not follow through with an exercise regime on their own. There's strength in numbers and you may need some extra support if you have any apprehension about exercise.

The right education regarding exercise and its benefits is important in helping develop the right attitude for a successful exercise plan. Try to forget past opinions and misconceptions about what you think exercise is all about. Do some research on the subject by talking to fitness professionals and gym members. They will point you in the right direction as to why they enjoy their program and how you can get started with one of your own. Many people from children to seniors have discovered the positive effects that exercise can provide.

Are you ready to give exercise a chance to change your life? It's very possible that once you let yourself make the same discovery you'll wonder why you didn't do it sooner. You'll be doing something very positive for yourself that will probably enhance the quality of the rest of your life.

Debra L. O'Melia

Enjoying the Gym Experience

I thought I would start with a list of some of the top excuses *not* to go to the gym.

1)   "I have no time." Think of your workout as something that you have to find time to do, just like working or running errands. If you stop to think about it, I'm sure you'd be surprised at how many hours in the week you waste doing other things that are a lot less important.

2)   "I can't afford a membership." Many gyms offer payment plans and specials. If your budget is really tight, then at least start walking or borrow some beginner workout videos from the library.

3)   "I'm too tired." Getting in a little cardio boost will wake you up, and the stimulating activity should help you sleep better too.

4)   "I don't have a babysitter." Most gyms offer child care for a small fee. If you can't afford it, then trade babysitting time with a friend or another member, and you can both save money.

5)   "I don't want to go alone." As soon as you walk in the door, you won't be alone. You may even make

new friends who would like to work out at the same time as you.

6) "Exercise will make me hungry." Exercising actually helps to control your appetite.

7) "I don't like to exercise." You obviously haven't given it a chance.

8) "I'll look silly." Well maybe you will, but just think about how you'll look at your next party or class reunion!

It was a big step for me to join a gym. I decided I had waited long enough and that this time I was going to make things work for me. There I was, ready to start my new adventure into the world of exercise. I walked into the gym knowing that I would probably be the heaviest woman there, and I was. Looking very chic in my size 5x jogging pants and my husband's old 6x T-shirt (we do try to conceal, don't we?), I began with a walk on the treadmill. Practically immobilized with fear, I held on with a death grip and refused to go any faster than a slow crawl. As I attempted to walk off my big caloric intake of the day, I tried to remember why I was there and why I was doing this. That's what you should be doing too. Remain focused on yourself. Don't get distracted by looking around trying to guess how much more or less you weigh than the other women. Don't worry about what they're thinking. You're not there for their benefit, you're there for yours. When you walk into the fitness center, leave the rest of the world outside and lavish your complete attention on yourself. This is your workout and you will get out what you put into it. Get into a place in your mind where you put yourself first. Whether you're working out at a health facility, walking in the park, or using an exercise video in your living room, this is *your* time; make the most of it. Always set regular portions of that time into your week, every week. If you do your best to keep your efforts at a steady pace, your results will appear sooner and your motivation will be stronger.

After a few weeks, I mastered my phobia of the treadmill. I was now ready to advance to the alien environment of the aerobics floor. I started out with muscle conditioning, which involves specific exercises with and without the use of free weights. I began with light weights and gradually worked my way up as my endurance increased. Muscle conditioning is an excellent way to burn fat and build lean muscle, which helps to firm and tone the body. This class is especially good for beginners because it is usually taught at a slower pace than other styles of exercise. Ask the staff to show you how to use some of the weight machines as well and add these to your workout. Don't worry about getting bulky. You're not going to end up looking like a body builder, but you may end up looking like someone who has nicely built up their body.

I then moved to the next phase on my agenda which was to try out an aerobics class. At first it was like being in a boring and repetitive dance class (Hey, I wanted to burn fat, not audition for a Broadway show!). I decided to give it a chance and gradually learned how to make the classes work for me. At times I felt ridiculous, but after a while I didn't care what I looked like doing this stuff called aerobics. Once I understood how it all worked, I began to enjoy and appreciate the benefits of cardiovascular exercise. When you first start your cardio program, begin with low impact sessions and work at your own level. Never try to keep up with anyone in the class. Your instructor will show you the proper modifications and monitor you during class. Always keep some water nearby to prevent dehydration. If you start to feel light-headed or short of breath, sit down and take a break until you feel that you can resume your workout. As a beginner you may not be able to complete an entire class. The important thing is that you showed up and you tried. Remember... start at your own pace and build up from there. My biggest challenge was step class. Step aerobics involves balancing yourself on a platform while attempting to perform various moves that are called out by the instructor. I tried to look graceful and stay in time with the rest of the class, but I was very uncoordinated and took a very long time to get my act together. However, once I did get everything to fall into place, step became my favorite class. If your gym offers step clinics I would suggest that you attend a few sessions before joining the more advanced students. Doing so may not only boost your confidence and lessen your frustration, but may also help to prevent injury by teaching you the proper techniques before you venture out on your own.

If you liked your class, remember to thank your instructor. She will appreciate the feedback. Teaching an exercise class is not as easy as it may seem. A competent instructor must not only teach the correct body mechanics and choreography, but she also has to remain aware of how everyone is feeling and performing. She has to keep the flow of the class steady, as well as keep track of the tempo of the music and the timing of the routine. On top of all this, she has to attempt to maintain a fun and interesting class for all of her students. When you think about all this, it will give you a real understanding of what goes into planning a good class. The instructor is the leader and is in charge the entire time that the class is in session. Once the music has started and her program begins, that is the signal that it is time to center on her and pay attention. Listen to the commands of your instructor. It may take some practice to get your timing where it should be. Eventually everything will fall into place and you'll probably forget just how awkward you may have been when you first started. Never hesitate to ask the staff questions if you are not sure of something you would like to try. They are there to help you.

Remember to have fun during all of your classes. Use the music to enhance your motivation and make every movement count during your routine. Maintain a positive attitude about what you are doing. As you become more proficient in your technique your enjoyment will increase and your attitude during class should show that. Let yourself go and revel in the good things that are happening to your body. With your heart rate climbing, endorphins surging, and your breathing steady and strong, you might even feel the urge to shout out your elation in front of the whole class. Don't be shy... go right ahead and yell! It's a compliment to your instructor and also shows that you have arrived as an accomplished member of the exercise arena.

Some Tips for Earning Positive Gains from Your Workout

To get the most from your program, it is important to understand what exercise can do for you. Consistency is key to a successful exercise formula. Remember to concentrate on what you are doing and why you are doing it. Work all major muscle groups using the proper form and safe amount of weight. Hold abdominal muscles in firmly to support lower back and always keep knees slightly bent when doing standing exercises. Stretching and warming up are just as important as the rest of your workout. Remember air and water. Your body needs a steady flow of oxygen and must stay well hydrated. Inhale through your nose and exhale through your mouth to maintain optimum air supply. You should drink plenty of water during exercise, so get into the habit of bringing a bottle of water with you. Wear appropriate footwear that is comfortable but provides adequate support. If you're not sure what to choose, get some advice from the gym. Don't overwork your body. Just like eating too little, exercising too much can cause your body to resist. Weight loss at a standstill? Try a little cross-training as a way of switching gears to jolt your body out of its metabolic "rut." For example, if you've been doing a lot of muscle work, take a break for a few days and switch to aerobics or more time on the treadmill. You may even want to consider some yoga classes to relieve stress and improve your flexibility. Like your nutritional program, your exercise skills will improve as your experience grows.

Enhancing Your Outward Appearance

What is your beauty trademark? What beauty signature do you show when you look in the mirror? The more important question is, do you show yours off the way you should, or do you allow yourself to just blend into the background? How do you measure beauty? Who are some of the people in your life that you consider beautiful? When the topic of beautiful women is mentioned, do you include yourself in that group? Do you make the most of what you have and enjoy who you are? You don't have to look like a runway model, but it would be nice to have a daily regime of beauty care. Women have no more excuses. Even men are using all sorts of beauty products to improve their looks. I'm not advocating turning yourself into what some people think is beautiful. I want you to create a look that is beautiful for *you*. If you're not satisfied with what you see in the mirror, then transform yourself, but do it in such a way that makes you happy, and create your own version of beautiful.

For years I didn't care about how I looked, and it showed. Once I started to gain weight, I lost all interest in my appearance. People who knew me back then tell me now how terrible I looked. With the combination of my excessive weight, round face and hair pulled straight back into a tight pony tail, I resembled a female version of a sumo wrestler. I paid no attention to anything that involved making me look more attractive. In my mind, I had no reason to put any effort into being more attractive or stylish. I was much more interested in putting all my energy into planning my next meal. Looking terrible and feeling depressed, I had now created the worst version of myself that I had ever experienced in my life! We all know that our problems will not be solved with a new hairstyle, different shade of lipstick or new wardrobe. However, all these things are a great boost to your self-image, and that is important in helping to maintain your motivation while you are working on other aspects of your plan. The results are immediate and can make a difference when you're in a slump with your long-term improvements.

If you've been following your fitness plan, your skin is probably enjoying and showing some of the benefits. Healthier eating, proper fluid intake, improved circulation and better sleeping habits can all help to revive the skin's tone and texture. Once you have worked at your skin from the inside, you'll have a better complexion to pamper on the outside. Now that you are drinking more water (you are, aren't you?), remember to also provide moisture from the outside as well. Always use cleansing products that are appropriate for your skin type. Don't use harsh soaps, and try to avoid using very warm water. Tepid or cool water is better, especially for the face. Exfoliates and facial scrubs are good to get rid of dead surface cells, but don't overuse them. It is a good idea to seek the advice of a dermatologist or other specialist if you have problems with your skin. Use of a moisturizer is particularly important after cleansing the face, at bedtime, and before a makeup application. Don't use anything that will clog your pores. Your skin is a living thing; it needs to breathe. Always use the proper sunscreen, and your skin will thank you in the future.

Healthy looking hair always plays a major role in a woman's appearance. Well maintained hair may seem like a little thing, but it can make a big difference about how you feel especially if you need a little motivation while going through your plan. A new hairstyle can be a nice quick fix if you need a little boost. Always start with a good cut that flatters your face. It's a good idea to see a professional stylist and choose something that you can easily duplicate and maintain. Like you skin, your hair needs gentle cleansing and adequate moisture. Get some professional advice on the best shampoo and conditioning agents for your hair type and use them consistently. Along with a new cut, think about adding some color or highlights that complement and accentuate your complexion and your features. It's the new you, so be daring and have fun.

Nail care is sometimes overlooked as part of the beauty routine. It's a nice touch to have well groomed nails, and to achieve this you have several choices. You can do your own nail care or look to a professional salon. Ask around to find a good one that will keep an eye on your nails' reactions to their products. Many women love the convenience of a salon treatment, but do-it-yourself home supplies are available. Go to a good beauty supply store for advice or ask someone who is experienced in nail care techniques. You'll not only have beautiful nails, but keeping your hands busy might keep you from reaching for those doughnuts or potato chips! If you're in the mood, don't forget to treat yourself to a nice pedicure as well. It'll be a nice reward for losing those five pounds.

Wearing makeup is, of course, a personal choice. If you've never experimented with cosmetics, give them a try because they can really help to play up your best features. Have fun and treat yourself to a free makeover at your local department store. The makeup artist can advise you about which skin care products and makeup shades will work best for you. The right combination of foundation, blush, lipstick and eye shadow can create a dramatic effect. Even a small detail like matching your nail polish to your lipstick creates a nicely coordinated look. Develop your own style to complement your wardrobe, the season or time of day.

Wear clothes that fit well. Trying to squeeze into a smaller size than what you really are is pointless. You'll look and feel much better if you stay true to your proper size. Accentuate the positive features about your figure while drawing attention away from what you don't like. If you were an overweight child or adolescent, you probably remember those lovely fashions that we were stuck wearing. When I was in school, I had to shop in a department called "CHUBETTE." The boys were sent to the land of the "HUSKY." What a wonderful way to boost a child's self-esteem! I just loved those stylish little A-line dresses. Fortunately, women and men now have a much better selection to choose from. A little careful shopping goes a long way in creating a great look that will make you feel confident and stylish.

Debra L. O'Melia

Some Advice on Cosmetic and

Reconstructive Surgery

Advances in cosmetic and reconstructive surgery have made procedures safer and more effective, but it is still a highly personal and individualized choice for any potential patient and should be approached with the utmost consideration and diligence. Considering these options is not just about vanity. It's about feeling good about yourself and your body image. After losing large amounts of weight, many women find that their body proportions are out of balance or they may have excess amounts of tissue that can only be corrected through surgery. This type of surgery should be treated as seriously as any other. You need to make sure that the surgeon that you choose has the proper skills, especially when you are contemplating fine work such as facial augmentation. Your regular physician can offer some suggestions or recommend certain licensing boards that may be able to match you with the appropriate specialist.

Word of mouth also seems to be a popular way to get information on the subject. It's great if you can actually get a chance to speak with a patient of your doctor of choice. This will enable you to get information on their handiwork and attention to detail. Avoid asking "How much?" Only the doctor can give you the bottom line. The doctor and their staff will judge the price after your initial consultation. They will evaluate how much of the doctor's time will be needed to complete the procedure and also calculate how much time they will need to reserve in the operating room if one is required.

Up to now, I have only been able to have one procedure performed. It was an abdominoplasty to correct a damaged abdominal wall caused by pregnancy and years of obesity. I was constantly being asked when I was "due." Although it was one of the more drastic procedures available, it made a world of difference in my appearance and made me feel more comfortable physically. My surgeon came highly recommended and I would not hesitate planning further procedures in the future.

Part Three

Debra L. O'Melia

Adapting to Your Grand Metamorphosis

Well here you are, all improved and transformed. Now what? How will life be after becoming a new person? You are about to begin a new phase of your life. How will you manage your life? What will you do differently? Will you look at yourself and the world in a different way? The image that you project may now be more confident and assertive. You will feel better and look better, and that should be reflected in how you present yourself to the world. Don't try to be everything to everybody. Just be the best you can be for yourself. In many ways you are still the same person. Don't change so much that you become someone that nobody knows anymore, including yourself. Some women cannot cope with the added attention or newfound interest in their new image. As a result their behavior becomes less than appealing and they find themselves in a place that is not good for them. Keep your feet on the ground and your destination in sight. Remember why you have done all of this and where you want to go from here.

Get ready to handle the reactions of others along the way. You may now command more respect. Some people will look at you differently, and take you more seriously. This is unfortunate because they should have been treating you that way in the first place. Some people that may have shunned you when you were heavier may gravitate towards you now. Still others may resent your startling alteration. In any case, you need to maintain a confidence in yourself and not worry about what others think. Losing a large amount of weight can bring many physical changes. You can feel parts of your body start to change shape. You may rediscover bones that hadn't shown themselves in years and may take pleasure in things like the loss of a double chin. You can now fit more easily into places that you couldn't before. Even your wardrobe has more variety, and you might even find yourself enjoying walking by full-length mirrors. One of my favorite moments occurred when I was walking in a wind storm and was now light enough to be pushed by a strong gust.

Appreciate your accomplishments. What you have done to make changes in your life is something to be proud of. Realize your value. Learn how to self-evaluate, and don't let others dictate your worth. You don't need others to validate who you are. Don't sell yourself short. Give yourself the credit you deserve for making things happen.

Let Your Spirit Shine

I have found that my coming out of hiding into a new light has become possible through a reform of mind, body and spirit. I knew that I had insights and desires harboring themselves inside of me, but over the years filed them away in my mind like forgotten recipes or old photographs. I knew they were there, but after awhile I just couldn't see them anymore. I was throwing away precious fragments of myself and allowing bitterness and resentment to overshadow my weary spirit.

Inner beauty can manifest itself in many ways and on many different levels. It can be that contagious smile that is shared with a stranger or a kindness shown to someone who may not always deserve your courtesy. It can mean holding a child when no one else will or crossing society's boundaries to ease someone's pain. It can also arrive in the form of a new welcoming of other's feelings and opinions, or learning to be more patient or letting others have the last word. Trying something new or exploring the unknown can yield a great bounty of rejuvenation for the soul.

Celebrate the differences in yourself and be more open to the same in others. Spread joy around and it will eventually come back to you. Let the world enjoy who you are by showing your beauty in your talents, compassion, and your ability to show love and receive it as well. Set your imagination free and let yourself dream. Learn how to recognize hidden blessings and messages of hope by listening to your intuitive senses. Let yourself revisit the fantasy world of your childhood to rekindle your vital essence. Let those you love know how you feel. Don't wait for a special occasion… it may never come.

My life experiences have taught me to take nothing good for granted. They have encouraged me to find positives in difficult situations and rely on simple pleasures to provide comfort in times of trouble. My faith has been my greatest source of strength and has played a large role in my ability to find hope even in the darkest of moments. It has shielded me through many conflicts and has made me feel protected and empowered. Prayers do get answered. We just need to listen and watch for the signs.

I still have much to learn and more to experience. I have a new kind of hunger and I look forward to the journey ahead. I need time to absorb all of my changes and experiences, both good and bad. I now look forward to the rest of my life and anticipate the joys of the future. I will try my best not to dwell on what I have lost but savor the beauty in life that I have gathered. I will take comfort in the love of my children and all of the special people in my life.

Love who you are and know what you can become and never let the journey end.

About the Author

Debra O'Melia makes her debut as an author with a practical guide to health and fitness. She delivers an enlightening and often personal look at the problems of obesity in a style of story telling that is sometimes humorous and at other times touching and thought provoking.

Her story includes an overview of her life as an obese child, adolescent and adult and how being overweight has effected her life. She also discusses how she has dealt with compulsive overeating and how it is possible to overcome an eating disorder with the right combination of understanding, determination and support.

Her book, *Royal Butterfly*, offers an example to those who are looking for a successful approach to weight loss and overall self-improvement.